5-Ingredient or Less Instant Pot Mediterranean Diet Cookbook 2020

The Simple Instant Pot Recipe Cookbook for Mediterranean Dieters to Live a Better Lifestyle, Cut Cooking Time and Save Money

By Coggin James

© Copyright 2020 – Coggin James- All rights reserved.

In no way is it legal to reproduce, duplicate, or transmit any part of this document by either electronic means or in printed format. Recording of this publication is strictly prohibited, and any storage of this material is not allowed unless with written permission from the publisher. All rights reserved.

Contents

Introduction..7

Chapter 1: Essentials Of Instant Pot Cooking...8

What Is An Instant Pot?..8

Types Of Instant Pot...8

Is An Instant Pot Safe?...9

How Does An Instant Pot Work?..9

Interesting Facts About Instant Pot..10

    Comes With An Amazing Sauté Feature... 10

    A Liquid Is Necessary To Cook.. 10

    Always Put The Pasta On Top... 11

    It Tends To Curdle Milk.. 11

    Allow It To Depressurize By Itself.. 11

    Yes, You Can Cook Frozen Meat... 11

    It Is Easy To Clean... 11

Chapter 2: Essentials Of Mediterranean Diet.. 12

What Is The Mediterranean Diet?... 12

Foods To Eat (How To Follow Mediterranean Diet).. 12

Foods To Avoid.. 13

Myths And Facts Of The Mediterranean Diet... 13

Health Benefits Of The Mediterranean Diet... 13

Chapter 3: Breakfast Recipes.. 14

    Mediterranean Egg Cups With Tomatoes... 14

    Milky Bulgur... 15

    Mediterranean Strawberry Oats.. 16

    Delightful Mediterranean Breakfast Oats... 17

    Egg Scramble With Greens... 18

    Instant Pot Horta And Potatoes.. 19

    Instant Pot Yellow Rice..20

    Instant Pot Yoghurt..21

Instant Pot Quinoa.. 22

Mediterranean Yellow Rice.. 23

Chapter 4: Soups, Stews, And Broths Recipes.. 24

Italian Beef Stew.. 24

Instant Pot Italian Chicken Stew... 25

Instant Pot Italian Beef Stew... 26

One-Pot Easy Beef Stew.. 27

Instant Pot Beef Stew With Sage And Red Wine... 28

Instant Pot Italian Sausage And Bean Soup.. 29

Instant Pot Crumbled Italian Sausage Soup.. 30

Instant Pot French Soup.. 31

Instant Pot French Onion Soup.. 32

Instant Pot Greek Lemon Chicken Soup.. 33

Chapter 5: Red Meat Recipes... 34

Instant Pot Beef Gyros With Tzatziki Sauce.. 34

Instant Pot Mississipi Roast Gyros... 35

Instant Pot Greek Beef Stew... 36

Beef Gyro... 37

Instant Pot Greek Lamb Beef Gyros.. 38

Pepperoncini Italian Beef.. 39

Easy Instant Pot Italian Beef... 40

Instant Pot Italian Beef... 41

Instant Pot Easy Italian Beef... 42

Instant Pot Sweet And Spicy Meatballs.. 43

Chapter 6: Poultry Recipes... 44

Instant Pot Turkey Stuffed Sweet Potatoes.. 44

Instant Pot Chicken Thighs With Sun-Dried Tomatoes And Artichokes........... 45

Instant Pot Mediterranean Turkey Cutlets.. 46

Instant Pot Mediterranean Chicken.. 47

- Instant Pot Mediterranean Chicken And Rice Bowl 48
- Instant Pot Sweet And Spicy Meatballs 49
- Instant Pot Chicken And Sweet Potatoes 50
- Duck And Veggies 51
- Mediterranean Whole Chicken 52
- Instant Pot Mediterranean Pasta Chicken 53

Chapter 7: Fish And Seafood 54
- Mediterranean Instant Pot Frozen Salmon 54
- Instant Pot Salmon 55
- Instant Pot Salmon With Rosemary 56
- Mediterranean Style Instant Pot Cod 57
- Clean Eating Mediterranean Rosemary Salmon 58
- Instant Pot Mediterranean Fresh Cod 59
- Instant Pot Cod And Peas With Sour Cream 60
- Instant Pot Delicious Lobster 61
- Instant Pot Sweet And Sour Fish 62
- Mediterranean Instant Pot Steamed Crab Legs 63

Chapter 8: Vegan And Vegetarian Recipes 64
- Instant Pot Black Eyed Peas 64
- Instant Pot Fasolakia (Green Beans And Potatoes In Olive Oil) 65
- Nutritious Vegan Cabbage 66
- Instant Pot Horta And Potatoes 67
- Instant Pot Jackfruit Curry 68
- Instant Pot Collard Greens With Tomatoes 69
- Instant Pot Artichokes With Mediterranean Aioli 70
- Instant Pot Millet Pilaf 71
- Instant Pot Stuffed Sweet Potatoes 72
- Instant Pot Couscous And Vegetable Medley 73

Chapter 9: Snacks And Dessert Recipes ... 74
- Natillas De Leche (Spanish Custard) ... 74
- Instant Pot Oatmeal Jars ... 75
- Cream Catalana ... 76
- Frixuelos De Asturias Recipe ... 77
- Instant Pot Yoghurt ... 78
- Easy Spanish Bread Pudding Recipe ... 79
- Peaches In Wine ... 80
- Instant Pot Italian Pasta ... 81
- Sweet And Salty Spanish Peanuts ... 82
- Instant Pot Chicken Shawarma ... 83

Conclusion ... 84

Appendix: Measurement Chart ... 85
- Liquid Volume Measurements ... 85
- Weight Conversions ... 85
- Liquid Volume Conversion ... 86
- Metric Temperature Conversions ... 86

Introduction

You have probably heard or read about the instant pot (IP). The instant pot is earning rave reviews online, and its fan base on Social media is growing immensely. Also, owing to its popularity, nowadays you can't read a food website or magazine without seeing an instant pot story.

If you don't own an Instant Pot, there is a good chance you have ordered one from Amazon.com, or you will receive one as a gift from a friend. The idea of getting your hands on this trendy multifunctional appliance generates reasonable curiosity and excitement, along with a dose of skepticism. I mean, how can one piece of equipment do the job of seven? How is an instant pot different from other multicookers?

A few years when I first heard about the instant pot, I did not understand how an appliance could combine the functions of a pressure cooker, slow cooker, Dutch oven, rice cooker, and more. After much use, I decided to save you the hassle and help you learn why an instant pot is worth a place on your kitchen counter.

The Instant Pot was designed to cut the number of hours spent in the kitchen. However, that has not been the case since most of the instant pot recipes are usually long. I have written this book to offer shorter alternatives to the time-consuming recipes. The entire book includes recipes that feature 5 or fewer ingredients. Each recipe is easy-to-follow, and anyone in your family can use the book to prepare delicious meals.

This book combines both Mediterranean Diet with Instant Pot cooking to help you live a easy Mediterranean life! Nowadays, too many people follow the Mediterranean Diet because of it's benefits given to followers! In this book, you will know all essentials about the Mediterranean Diet. And you will be happy with this amazing book!

Ready? Let's get started!

Chapter 1: Essentials of Instant Pot Cooking

What is an instant pot?

An Instant Pot is a 3rd generation programmable multicooker designed to do the job of a rice cooker, slow cooker, electric pressure cooker, steamer, sauté/browning pan, yogurt maker, and warming pot. It is an innovative kitchen appliance that rolls the functions of seven different appliances into one package.

The appliance features multiple preset programs that allow you to cook food to perfection. Want to cook rice? An instant pot will do that. Want to slow cook dinner? It will do that, too. The Instant Pot is a versatile appliance that seems way too good to be real.

The specific functions of an instant pot vary depending on the model your purchase. However, every Instant pot features some basic, preset programs which include:

- Rice cooker
- Pressure cooker (allows you to cook food on low or high pressure, or select specific pressure settings for meat or stew)
- Slow Cooker
- Sauté/Browning
- Steamer
- Warmer
- Yogurt Maker

Some Instant Pot models may include other functions such as cake maker, sterilizer, and egg maker. Additionally, the IP comes with a timer and other settings that enable you to set food to cook on low, medium, or high temperatures.

Types of Instant Pot

Instant Pot is a brand name owned by Instant Brands; a Canadian company founded in 2009 by technology gurus. The Instant Pot was introduced in 2010 after 18 months of rigorous research, development, and design. The first IP was the CSG Multi-Use Programmable Pressure Cooker; an innovative device that included the functions of 5 cooking appliances; pressure cooker, rice cooker, warmer, and steamer.

Over time the Instant Pot brand has evolved to about 20 unique models. The models range in size such as:

- 3-quarts: Perfect for small families (2 to 3 people)
- 5-quarts to 6-quarts: Ideal for medium sized families (4 to 6 people)
- 8-quarts: Ideal for large families (6 or more people)

Some of the popular Instant Pot models include:

- Max
- Ultra
- Duo
- Duo Plus
- Lux
- Nova

- Nova Plus
- Viva
- Smart Bluetooth

The Instant Pot Smart Bluetooth is a highly innovative model that allows you to control and monitor cooking from your mobile device (phone or tablet).

As you may notice, other renowned manufacturers such as Breville, Cuisinart, and Gourmia offer appliances that feature the functions of an Instant Pot. As a result, you will be spoilt to choice, when selecting your ideal appliance. So do your homework, and select an appliance that will best serve your needs.

Is an instant pot safe?

In the modern world, trendy appliances burst into the scene with glamor and glitz that conceal the underlying worries. There is no denying, the Instant Pot trend has gone viral, and the buzz is yet to settle. Because of this, it may be rare to find a consumer critiquing the safety of this popular item.

When I first got an Instant Pot, I was cautious about its use. Although the appliance seemed a game-changer and time-saver, I had qualms about how secure it was. I knew the instant pot is principally a programmable pressure cooker, and this further intensified my worries.

I mean, we have had numerous stories about pressure cooker exploding and hurting someone. So, are freak accidents involving Instant Pot covered? How much risk should one assume when using an Instant Pot?

If you have any worry about the use of an Instant Pot, trash the doubt. Unlike the pressure cookers used by our fore-parents in the 1980s, the Instant Pot is safe. Chances of the IP exploding are minimal as the device has no issues with overheating and melting.

The Instant Pot comes with several security features. For example, the IP comes with an automatic lid lock with detection features. This means it is impossible to open the lid until all the pressure has been released. Besides, the IP has an anti-blockage vent designed to ensure that particles of food do not block the steam vent. The automatic temperature control feature ensures the inside temperatures are within the safe range.

How does an instant pot work?

As aforementioned, the Instant Pot is primarily a programmable pressure cooker. To understand how this appliance works, you must first understand its architecture.

The Instant Pot is made of three major components; **the cover/lid, the inner pot, and the outer pot.** The three components work in unison to accelerate cooking.

- The **outer pot** accommodates the control panel, the heat source, the sensor (temperature & pressure), and the motherboard.
- On the other hand, the inner pot is housed inside of the outer pot. It is the place where the food being cooked is placed.
- The cover of the IP functions as the chief safety feature. The cover features the locking mechanism, pressure release valves, and the gaskets. It features an airtight seal that locks food in the inner pot creating the perfect cooking environment.

Now that you know the components of an Instant Pot, it should be easy for you to understand how it works.

There is no magic to how an instant pot works. When you select a cooking function on the control panel, the click of the button sends a signal to the IP's motherboard. The motherboard switches on the heat source which is located at the outside base of the inner pot. Because the cover is tightly sealed, the air inside the inner pot heats up rapidly, and the liquid in the pot also heats up turning into steam. This leads to increased pressure in the inner pot, which ultimately expedites cooking.

Now, the Instant Pot features a flexible plate housed underneath the heat source. The flexible plate bends to activate the pressure/temperature sensor when maximum tolerable pressure and temperatures are reached. The sensor sends a signal to the motherboard causing it to shut off the heat source.

Once the heat source is switched off, the pressure inside the inner pot drops. The flexible plate flattens out, and the pressure/temperature sensor is deactivated. A signal is sent to the motherboard, and the IP is switched on once more. This process of on/off cycles continues until the food being cooked is ready. The duration and number on/off heating cycles will depend on the cooking function selected on the control panel.

Interesting facts about Instant Pot

It's no surprise that the hottest kitchen appliance to land on your counter does so much when it comes to pressure cooking. This wonderful device has had a tremendous makeover, and now you can use it to sear meat, sauté vegetables, cook pasta- the possibilities are endless. It's referred to as a 7-in-one, and for a good reason – it can handle different cooking methods all in one gadget.

There are some important things you need to know before using this multitasker. Sure, this tool is going to save you loads of time and space in addition to cooking your food ridiculously fast. But if you're going to master this kitchen appliance, you need to know the basic and interesting facts about it.

Comes with an Amazing Sauté Feature

The Instant Pot has an incredible sauté feature that is often overlooked by many people. From its appearance, you wouldn't imagine that something that resembles a Crock Pot would do a great job of sautéing foods. But this gadget gives much more than an ordinary Crock Pot.

Pressing the sauté button on the instant pot automatically triggers the bottom of the pot to heat up, and you can sauté anything you want in the hot pan. This feature comes in handy when you want to sauté vegetables, brown or sear your meat before cooking, or make the soup that needs pasta. Whatever you do, make sure you use the sauté feature. It will do the magic.

A liquid is necessary to cook

Another important thing that people overlook is that liquid is needed to build the pressure to cook. If you plan to cook meat in the Instant Post, remember to add a minimum of one cup of liquid or it will fail to build the steam to cook.

The liquid can be either water, broth, or any other type of liquid that can create great steam for pressure cooking. Be careful not to use too much liquid as it may lead to loss of flavor. If you choose to use a thicker liquid, dilute it first to ensure it's able to create pressure for efficient cooking.

Always put the pasta on top

It's amazing how you can cook a variety of dishes -meat, pasta, sauce, everything in one pot. Most of the cooking methods cook pasta by submerging it into a liquid for even cooking. While it is important to do it this way when you're boiling a dish that contains pasta, it's different in a pressure cooker.

In the Instant Pot, always add the pasta noodles last, right on top. Immersing them in the liquid will likely end up with mushy noodles. Although they may still taste okay, we are not aiming for a yack meal, but a well-prepared pasta cooked under the right amount of pressure.

It tends to curdle milk

While it can do fantastic things in the kitchen, one of the drawbacks of cooking with the Instant Pot is that sometimes it tends to create a heat that's so high, to curdle any milk that may be used in the recipe. Curdling occurs when the proteins present in the milk separate.

Although the foods are perfectly safe to eat, they may not have the desired texture or taste that you want. You might consider using dairy-inclusive recipes that contain cheese, but it is important to test the different kinds of dairy and recipes to find out which one doesn't lead to this issue.

Allow it to depressurize by itself

When you're preparing your favorite beef ribs, a common mistake you can make is to manually vent it immediately for a quick release as soon as the cook cycle is over. The result is that the immediate change of temperature and pressure can make the meat to be very tough, which is not what you want.

Once you're done with the cooking, let the pot cool down for a while to release pressure naturally. You'll know the pressure has been released when you see the silver button drop down on top of the lid. This is known as the Natural Pressure Release (NPR). This setting is always used for meats unless you prefer dry meals for dinner.

Yes, you can cook frozen meat

The idea of putting frozen meat in a slow cooker is a nightmare to many people as the delicacy may be sitting at an unsafe temperature for too long. But with Instant Pot, you have more choices and freedom with the frozen meat. You don't have to defrost it before cooking it in the Instant Pot. You will need to increase your cook time by fifty percent, but it will cook the frozen meat perfectly well. Avoid using large roasts or thick pieces of frozen meat. In this case, we are referring to steaks, chicken breasts, meatballs, chicken thighs, and other thinner cuts of meat.

It is easy to clean

Who doesn't hate the tedious cleaning of dishes after cooking? I do, and I assume you do too. After spending hours in the kitchen to create a wonderful meal, the last thing you want to think about are the dishes.

The good news is that using Instant Pot save you the hustle of having to clean it. Soo much after use. It comes with an inner stainless-steel lining which is easily removable when you want to clean it. Usually, a small wipe down of the lid will do the magic, and it's all cleaned up and ready for the next cooking session.

Chapter 2: Essentials of Mediterranean Diet

What is the Mediterranean diet?
When you hear about the Mediterranean diet, what comes to your mind? The Greek lamb chops? Italian pasta and pizza? Lasagna? Or endless bottles of wine?

There is no denying; the Mediterranean diet is a broad diet that entails several cuisines draw from the Mediterranean region. The diet is popular in many parts of the world and is often regarded as one of the healthiest diets.

If you are looking to put your lifestyle back on to a healthier path, then this diet is worth chasing.

The Mediterranean diet is a super healthy diet practiced by communities living in the 21 countries that surround the Mediterranean Sea. It is a diet build around the traditional ingredients that the people living in the Mediterranean region used to consume.

The origin of this diet dates back in 1960, and although it's called a diet, it is not really a diet. It is a lifestyle that inspires people to consume healthy fast, plant-based foods, whole grains, and an occasional glass of wine. The diet is extensively embraced by medical experts, and research continues to unearth many of its health benefits.

As you may notice, the old-age habit of consuming a Mediterranean diet is deeply rooted in countries such as Spain, Egypt, Greece, Italy, France, and other northern Africa countries. Researchers found that people living in the Mediterranean region were remarkably healthy and showed little vulnerability to common lifestyle diseases.

Multiple studies have shown the numerous benefits of the Mediterranean diet. This has propelled the popularity of this diet, and it is no surprise that it is one of the widely practiced diet in the world.

Foods to Eat (How to Follow Mediterranean Diet)
The Mediterranean diet is based around eating vegetables, poultry, herbs & spice, eggs, fruits, nuts, olive oils, whole grains, legumes, nuts & seeds, tubers, and fish.

That said; you should note that the Mediterranean diet doesn't define the exact foods you should eat. There are glaring variations between the foods consumed in different Mediterranean countries, hence the controversy.

If you are looking to start a Mediterranean diet lifestyle, here are the key points to get you started:

- Increase the daily consumption of plant-based foods.
- Go for veggies
- Make the most of whole grains
- Add fruits to your diet plan
- Use legumes to cook hearty, meatless dishes and soups
- Spice up things with spices, seeds, and nuts
- Olive oil should be your only cooking oil

- Eating fish at least twice a week won't hurt
- Moderate the consumption of eggs and dairy products
- Reduce the consumption of red meat and increase that of poultry
- Drink red wine moderately
- Exercise regularly

Foods to Avoid

The foods to avoid when practicing a Mediterranean diet lifestyle include Trans fats, processed meat, refined oils, added sugar, refined grains, and processed foods.

Myths and Facts of the Mediterranean diet

Although the Mediterranean diet has been around for long, it is still riddled by numerous misconceptions. Here are some myths about the Mediterranean diet:

- **The diet is all about foods:**

Many people think the Mediterranean diet is only about foods. Even though the food is the biggest pillar of this diet, embracing the way of life of the Mediterraneans is pivotal. Also, doing regular physical activities is as important as what you put on your plate.

- **Eating huge amounts of pasta and bread is okay:**

As you may notice, communities in the Mediterranean region do not eat large bowls of pasta as the Americans do. Pasta and bread are usually side dishes, and the Mediterraneans do not take them as main dishes.

- **Mediterranean diet is expensive**

The ingredients of a Mediterranean diet are readily available in the grocery store. Also, compared to other diets, the Mediterranean diet focuses on plant-based ingredients such as lentil or beans, which make it less expensive.

Health benefits of the Mediterranean diet

As mentioned earlier, the Mediterranean diet offers numerous health benefits. Studies have found that people who practice the Mediterranean way of life experience incredible health benefits. Some of the notable benefits of the Mediterranean diet include:

- Mediterranean diet reduces the risk of heart diseases such as myocardial infarction, stroke, and cardiovascular disease.
- It prevents cognitive decline and preserves memory.
- It helps control blood sugar and manage diabetes.
- It helps fight depression
- It strengthens bones
- It protects against cancer.

Chapter 3: Breakfast Recipes

MEDITERRANEAN EGG CUPS WITH TOMATOES

These are awesomely delicious healthy egg cups which are very easy to prepare and fit for every member of your family. The cups can be carried to work in your lunchbox or as a snack. Make them in advance and store in the freezer then just heat in your microwave in the morning.

TIME: 35 MINUTES | **SERVING:** 2

INGREDIENTS

2 tomatoes

3/4 Black pepper (ground)

1 tbsp dill (Fresh and chopped)

1/4 tbsp paprika

2 eggs

METHOD

1. Cut the tomatoes huts then remove the flesh.
2. Mix pepper, dill, and paprika in a small mixing bowl. Place the mixture in the tomato cup.
3. Beat the egg in the cups and wrap the cups in a foil. Place them on your instant pot bowl.
4. Lid and set time for fifteen minutes on high. Release pressure naturally for ten minutes.
5. Remove the tomatoes from the instant pot then remove tomatoes carefully from foil. Discard the foil.
6. Serve and enjoy.

NUTRITIONAL INFORMATION

Cal: 97 | Fat: 8g | Carbs: 1.1g | Fiber: 0.4g | Protein: 5.9g | Sugar: 0g

MILKY BULGUR

This is a fantastic tasting Mediterranean milky bulgur made right from your instant pot. Put the ingredients in your instant pot, and in some few minutes, a hearty breakfast is on the table. This milky bulgur kicks off your day in high spirits.

TIME: 20 MINUTES | **SERVING:** 4

INGREDIENTS

1 cup bulgur

2 tbsp sugar

1 tbsp vanilla extract

2 cups milk

1 tbsp butter

METHOD

1. Place the bulgur in your instant pot bowl. Add sugar, vanilla, and milk.
2. Lid the instant pot and set time for 6 minutes on high. Pressure release quickly then remove the bulgur from the instant pot.
3. Add butter then stir.
4. Serve and enjoy.

NUTRITIONAL INFORMATION

Cal: 232 | Fat: 5.9g | Carbs: 38.7g | Fiber: 6.4g | Protein: 8.3g | Sugar: 0g

MEDITERRANEAN STRAWBERRY OATS

This is a sweet, tangy strawberry oat. The high fiber content keeps you full for a long time or until the next meal. The fresh strawberries make them kids lovers. Try these oats in your instant pot since they are really easy to prepare.

TIME: 20 MINUTES | **SERVING:** 4

INGREDIENTS

1 cup oats (rolled)

2 cups water

1 tbsp honey

1 tbsp coconut flakes

1/2 Cup strawberries (chopped)

METHOD

1. Place the oats in the instant pot. Pour water and close the instant pot lid.
2. Set time for five minutes on high pressure. When the time has elapsed release pressure quickly and transfer the cooked oats in a bowl.
3. Add honey and stir. Sprinkle coconut flakes and strawberries.
4. Serve and enjoy.

NUTRITIONAL INFORMATION

Cal: 134| Fat: 2g| Carbs: 26.2g| Fiber: 33g| Protein: 3.8g| Sugar: 0g

DELIGHTFUL MEDITERRANEAN BREAKFAST OATS

Do you have an instant pot in your kitchen? If the answer is yes, then these delightful and insanely addictive breakfast oats are worth a trial. They are delicious, easy, filling for a long time and cheap to prepare right from your home.

TIME: 15 MINUTES | **SERVING:** 4

INGREDIENTS

8 oz. oats (rolled)

1 tbsp butter

1 tbsp vanilla extract

1 tbsp honey

1 oz. walnuts (crushed)

METHOD

1. Place the oats in your instant pot then add butter, vanilla and two cups of milk. Stir well then lid your instant pot
2. Set time to five minutes on medium pressure. When time is done release the pressure quickly.
3. Share the oats among the serving bowls. Add honey and walnuts on each bowl.
4. Serve and enjoy.

NUTRITIONAL INFORMATION

Cal: 347 | Fat: 11.3g | Carbs: 49.6g | Fiber: 6.2g | Protein: 13.2g | Sugar: 0g

EGG SCRAMBLE WITH GREENS

This is awesomely delicious scrambled eggs that you can make in your instant pot. The eggs are very easy to prepare, cheap, and quite satisfying until the next meal. These eggs are kids' favorite and are rich in nutrients, so it is healthy to take more often.

TIME: 40 MINUTES | **SERVINGS:** 4

INGREDIENTS

1 tbsp olive oil

1/4 Cup cilantro and spinach each (fresh and chopped)

1 oz. parsley (chopped)

Salt and white pepper to taste

4 eggs

METHOD

1. Pour oil in your instant pot. Add cilantro, spinach, parsley, salt, and pepper then stir them. Sauté for about five minutes.
2. Meanwhile, whisk the eggs in a mixing bowl and pour the eggs on the greens.
3. Continue to sauté for two minutes then scramble the sautéed eggs. Lid and cook for twelve minutes on high pressure.
4. Release the pressure naturally then remove the eggs from the instant pot.
5. Serve and enjoy.

NUTRITIONAL INFORMATION

Cal: 97 | Fat: 8g | Carbs: 1.1g | Fiber: 0.4g | Protein: 5.9g | Sugar: 0g

INSTANT POT HORTA AND POTATOES

This amazing Horta and potatoes is a Hit in most Mediterranean living. So grab your instant pot and let your family enjoy this healthy and delicious dish. It's now easy to make, and in a matter of a few minutes, it will ready.

TIME: 25 MINUTES | **SERVINGS:** 4

INGREDIENTS

2 greens head (kale, spinach, dandelion, mustard greens, Swiss chard) thoroughly washed, chopped.

6 potatoes (washed and cut in pieces)

1 cup virgin olive oil

1 lemon juice (preserve slices for serving)

10 garlic cloves (chopped)

METHOD

1. Pour all the ingredients in the instant pot. Add a cup of water, salt, and pepper to taste then stir well.
2. Lid the instant pot and set the vent to sealing. Set time for fifteen minutes .when time has elapsed release the pressure.
3. Remove the Horta and potatoes from the instant pot and let cool.
4. Serve and enjoy with lemon slices.

NUTRITIONAL INFORMATION

Cal: 69.7 | Fat: 5.5g | Carbs: 4.6g | Fiber: 2g | Protein: 1.7g | Sugar: 0.9g

INSTANT POT YELLOW RICE

This is a real recreate from your favorite restaurant meal. It may be a dinner leftover taken for breakfast or cooked afresh in the morning for a heavy breakfast. It's quite filling and very easy to prepare in those busy mornings.

TIME: 10 MINUTES | **SERVING:** 6

INGREDIENTS

2 cups stock (chicken)

1/2 tbsp turmeric

1 bay leaf

1 cup rice (long grain)

1 tbsp butter (unsalted)

METHOD

1. Rinse your long grain rice until the water runs clear.
2. Pour the rice in the instant pot followed by all other ingredients except butter. Stir until the rice is evenly distributed.
3. Lid the instant pot and set time for three minutes.
4. Allow a natural release of pressure. Remove the lid then add butter. Use a fork to fluff the rice.
5. Serve and enjoy.

NUTRITIONAL INFORMATION

Cal: 158 | Fat: 3g | Carbs: 27g | Fiber: 0g | Protein: 4g | Sugar: 1g

INSTANT POT YOGHURT

Are you a yogurt lover but the price is really discouraging? I hope your answer is yes. This homemade yogurt is cheaper, creamier and very easy to prepare. So make yogurt from your home and quench that sweet craving in the morning.

TIME: 9 HOURS 30 MINUTES | **SERVING:** 8 CUPS

INGREDIENTS

8 cups whole milk

1/4 Cup whole milk yogurt (plain)

METHOD

1. Add milk in your instant pot insert and lid the instant pot.
2. Select the yogurt function on the instant pot and boil up to an hour.
3. Cool the instant pot in ice cold water for twenty minutes. Set aside a cup of milk.
4. Pour yogurt in mixing bowl and whisk together with the reserved milk. Stir in the mixture into the remaining milk ensuring you don't scrap the insert bottom.
5. Set time for eight hours.
6. When time is done transfer the yogurt into storage jars for refrigeration up to ten days.
7. Serve and enjoy.

NUTRITIONAL INFORMATION

Cal: 89 | Fat: 11g | Carbs: 9g | Fiber: 0g | Protein: 20g | Sugar: 9g

INSTANT POT QUINOA

Are you a quinoa lover? Do you own an instant pot? An instant pot makes the perfect quinoa. It's easy, fluffy and very addictive. It drives hunger away and is fit for every member of your family.

TIME: 20 MINUTES | **SERVING:** 6

INGREDIENTS

2 cups quinoa

1 tbsp avocado oil

1 onion (diced)

1 tbsp garlic (minced)

2.5 cups vegetable broth

METHOD

1. Soak your quinoa in water for an hour and place on a metal strainer.
2. Rinse with cold water until water is clear.
3. Turn on the sauté function on your instant pot. Add oil and onions then stir cook. Add minced garlic followed by quinoa then sauté for five more minutes.
4. Add broth and salt and pepper to taste then lid the instant pot.
5. Set time for one minute at high pressure. When time is done naturally release the pressure.
6. Remove lid and remove quinoa from the instant pot.
7. Serve and enjoy.

NUTRITIONAL INFORMATION

Cal: 242 | Fat: 5g | Carbs: 39g | Fiber: 4g | Protein: 8g | Sugar: 1g

MEDITERRANEAN YELLOW RICE

Have you tried rice on your instant pot? If no, then you really are missing out. This Mediterranean instant pot yellow rice leftover makes a perfectly delicious filling breakfast for you and your family.

TIME: MINUTES | **SERVING:** 4

INGREDIENTS

1 cup white rice

1.5 cups broth or water

Salt and pepper

1/8 tbsp turmeric

1/4 tbsp garlic powder

METHOD

1. Put all the ingredients in the instant pot and briefly stir them.
2. Lid the Instant pot and set the vent at sealing. Set the rice function at twelve minutes on your instant pot.
3. When the time has elapsed release pressure naturally then fluff the rice using a fork.
4. Serve and enjoy.

NUTRITIONAL INFORMATION

Cal: 170 | Fat: 0.3g | Carbs: 37.2g | Fiber: 0.6g | Protein: 3.3g | Sugar: 0.1g

Chapter 4: Soups, Stews, and Broths Recipes

ITALIAN BEEF STEW

This is a delicious beef stew to make in your instant pot. Beef is a rich source of iron which is essential for red blood cells to transport oxygen in the body's cells. Thus this beef stew is a very healthy Mediterranean recipe.

TIME: 45 MINUTES | **SERVINGS:** 6

INGREDIENTS

2 lbs. stew meat

1 tbsp olive oil

Spices: 1(6 oz.) can tomato paste, 4 tbsp minced garlic, 1/2 cup balsamic vinegar

Veggies: 1/2 cup chopped onion, 4 red potatoes (1-inch pieces), 3 peeled carrots (half cut), sprigs of rosemary and thyme oregano

3 cups beef broth

METHOD

1. Turn your instant pot to sauté mode then add olive oil till it's hot.
2. Add the stew meat in one layer and brown it.
3. Add all others ingredients, stir and seal the pot. Turn to stew/meat mode.
4. Cook for about 35 minutes then release pressure naturally.
5. Unseal the pot and stir while adjusting salt for desired taste.
6. Serve and enjoy!

NUTRITIONAL INFORMATION

Calories: 406 | Fat: 10g | Carbs: 37g | Protein: 39g | Sodium: 844mg | Potassium: 1710mg

INSTANT POT ITALIAN CHICKEN STEW

This is a fantastic chicken stew to prepare in the instant pot. The stew has shredded and tender chicken along with vegetables. It is a low carb, paleo, keto, and gluten-free Mediterranean recipe.

TIME: 55 MINUTES | **SERVINGS:** 4

INGREDIENTS

12 ounces chicken thighs (boneless and skinless)

2 tbsp olive oil

Spices: 14 ounces tomatoes (diced and unsalted), 1 tbsp tomato paste, 1 tbsp salt, 1/2 tbsp dried oregano, 1/2 tbsp pepper

Veggies: 2 bay leaves, 1/2 chopped onion, 2 stalks chopped celery, 1 chopped carrot, 1/2 cup kalamata olives (chopped and pitted), 1/2 cup chopped basil leaves (fresh and loosely packed)

$1\frac{1}{2}$ cups chicken broth (low sodium)

METHOD

1. Turn your instant pot to sauté mode for medium heat then add oil to the pot.
2. Once hot, add onion, carrot, and celery then cook for about 5 minutes while stirring to soften them.
3. Add the diced tomatoes with the liquid, basil, chicken broth, bay leaves, tomato paste, oregano, pepper, and salt.
4. Stir for the tomato paste to dissolve then turn off sauté mode.
5. Add the chicken thighs (make sure they are covered by the liquid). Seal the pot.
6. Cook for about 10 minutes under high pressure then release pressure naturally for about 10 minutes. Quick release the rest.
7. Unseal the pot, transfer the chicken to a plate and turn on sauté mode for low heat.
8. Meanwhile, shred the chicken with 2 forks.
9. Return the shredded chicken to the pot then add kalamata olives.
10. Simmer for about 10 minutes while occasionally stirring to get desired stew consistency.
11. Serve hot.

NUTRITIONAL INFORMATION

Calories: 230 | Fat: 15g | Carbs: 10.5g | Proteins: 16g | Sodium: 390mg | Potassium: 80mg

INSTANT POT ITALIAN BEEF STEW

This is a colorful, hearty, and a nourishing Mediterranean beef stew. It is an instant pot dish that is easy to prepare, and everyone in your family will love it.

TIME: 35 MINUTES | **SERVINGS:** 6

INGREDIENTS

1 lb. beef stew meat

1 tbsp olive oil

Liquids: 2 cups water, 1 (32 oz.) can beef broth,

Veggies: 1 diced white onion, 2 minced garlic cloves, 4 sliced carrots, 3 sliced celery stalks, 10 red potatoes (small quartered), 3 sprigs of oregano, 4-6 basil leaves,

Spices: 2 ($14\frac{1}{2}$ oz) cans stewed tomatoes (drained), 2 tbsp salt, 2 tbsp pepper

METHOD

1. Turn your instant pot to sauté mode until hot.
2. Add olive oil, garlic, onions, and beef stew meat. Cook while constantly stirring. Make sure the beef gets seared all sides.
3. Turn off sauté mode then add celery, potatoes, carrots, and the stewed tomatoes.
4. Add the liquids making sure the max fill line is not exceeded. Top with basil leaves, oregano, pepper and salt and stir well.
5. Seal the pot and cook for about 20 minutes under high pressure then quick release pressure.
6. Serve along with garlic bread.

ONE-POT EASY BEEF STEW

This one-pot easy beef stew is absolutely a comfort dinner food. It is an instant pot dish that gives you all flavors of slow cooking in a fraction of time. It is a delicious Mediterranean recipe to try during the busy weeknights.

TIME: 55 MINUTES | SERVINGS: 5

INGREDIENTS

2.5 lb. beef chuck meat (fat trimmed and 2 inch cubes cut)

Spices: 2 tbsp kosher salt, 1 tbsp black pepper, 1/2 tbsp smoked paprika, 1 tbsp onion powder, 1 tbsp garlic powder, 1/4 tbsp cayenne pepper

Veggies: 1 diced onion, 1 shredded carrot

2 tbsp all-purpose flour

Liquids: 8-oz tomato sauce, 1/4 cup water

METHOD

1. Place beef chuck meat, spices, veggies, and all-purpose flour in the instant pot and stir to mix.
2. Add the liquids and stir again.
3. Seal the pot and cook for about 45 minutes under manual high pressure then release pressure naturally for about 15 minutes. Quick release the remaining pressure.
4. Serve warm.

NUTRITIONAL INFORMATION

Calories: 443 | Fat: 26g | Carbs: 8g | Protein: 44g | Sodium: 1362mg | Potassium: 981mg

INSTANT POT BEEF STEW WITH SAGE AND RED WINE

This is a delicious instant pot beef stew which is an adaption of Italian old traditional recipe. This is a very healthy dish since Beef is a rich source of iron which is essential for red blood cells to transport oxygen in the body's cells.

TIME: 35 MINUTES | **SERVINGS:** 4-8

INGREDIENTS

$1\frac{1}{2}$ pound stew beef (bite-size pieces)

1 tbsp olive oil (extra virgin)

Spices: $\frac{1}{2}$ tbsp salt, $\frac{1}{2}$ tbsp sage, 1 tbsp black pepper, 1 tbsp thyme,

Veggies: 1 chopped red pepper, 4 small potatoes (bite-size pieces), 2 thinly sliced zucchini, 10 oz. mushrooms

Liquids: $1\frac{1}{2}$ cup water, $1\frac{1}{2}$ cup red wine

METHOD

1. Turn instant pot to sauté mode.
2. Add beef stew and olive oil and sauté to brown the beef stew on all sides.
3. Add all the remaining ingredients, stir well and seal the pot.
4. Cook for about 20 minutes under manual high pressure then release pressure naturally. Unseal the pot
5. Serve immediately.

INSTANT POT ITALIAN SAUSAGE AND BEAN SOUP

The instant pot Italian sausage and bean soup is a stick-to-your-ribs type of soup. It is a Mediterranean soup that is hearty and very easy to prepare. Your family will absolutely love this recipe.

TIME: 20 MINUTES | **SERVINGS:** 8

INGREDIENTS

1-1$\frac{1}{2}$ lbs. bulk sausage

Veggies: 1 large chopped onion, 2 minced garlic cloves

2 tbsp dried basil

Shredded parmesan (for each bowl)

2 cans undrained butter beans

2 cans drained and rinsed black beans

2 cans diced tomatoes

2 cans beef broth

METHOD

1. Turn your instant to sauté mode.
2. Add sausage, garlic and onion then cook until sausage cooks through.
3. Darin grease then add other ingredients apart from parmesan cheese.
4. Seal the pot and cook for about 5 minutes then quick release pressure.
5. Divide among 8 bowls and top with the cheese.
6. Serve and enjoy!

INSTANT POT CRUMBLED ITALIAN SAUSAGE SOUP

This crumbled sausage soup is so satisfying and easy to make in the instant pot. It is a healthy Mediterranean recipe as sausages provide relief from fatigue and weakness.

TIME: 35 MINUTES | **SERVINGS:** 6

INGREDIENTS

1 pound mild Italian sausage (ground)

3 tbsp olive oil

Liquids: 1 cup water, 4 cups chicken stock,

Spices: 1 tbsp pepper, 2 tbsp salt

Veggies: 1 diced medium onion, 1 (15-ounce) can drained and rinsed navy beans, 1 ($14\frac{1}{2}$ ounce) can diced petite tomatoes, 1 cup chopped frozen spinach

1 cup pasta (short and dried)

$\frac{1}{2}$ Cup shredded parmesan

METHOD

1. Turn your instant pot to sauté mode until hot.
2. Add olive oil and sausage then cook for about 10 minutes until the sausage is browned. Drain and set aside.
3. Place onions in the pot and cook for about 3 minutes until translucent then carefully pour the chicken stock.
4. Add beans, spinach, pasta, tomatoes, water pepper, and salt. Stir and seal the pot.
5. Cook for about 5 minutes under manual high pressure then release pressure naturally for about 5 minutes.
6. Unseal the pot then add the cheese and stir.
7. Serve immediately.

INSTANT POT FRENCH SOUP

This is a fantastic instant pot French soup that will leave you yearning for more. It is a satisfying Mediterranean soup which is fabulous and delicious and is perfect for the chaotic weeknights.

TIME: 1 HOUR | **SERVINGS:** 8

INGREDIENTS

5 lb. thinly sliced yellow onion

1 tbsp olive oil

For broth: $\frac{1}{4}$ cup red wine, $\frac{1}{3}$ cup soy sauce, 2 tbsp Worcestershire sauce, 8 cups beef broth, 2 tbsp minced dry onions, $\frac{1}{2}$ tbsp dried oregano, $\frac{1}{4}$ tbsp dried thyme, 1 bay leaf, 1 tbsp minced garlic

For garnish: 8 slices French bread, 1 tbsp olive oil, $1\frac{1}{2}$ cups swiss gruyere, parmesan sprinkling

METHOD

1. Turn instant pot to sauté mode then add oil until heated up.
2. Add onion and sauté for about 3 minutes until fragrant then turn off sauté mode.
3. Add red wine and let it simmer. Deglaze the pan with a wooden spoon by scraping brown bits from the bottom.
4. Add the broth ingredients and seal the pot.
5. Cook for about 25 minutes under manual setting then quick release pressure.
6. Meanwhile, preheat an oven to 450°F with a sheet pan lined with a parchment paper.
7. Brush French bread on both sides with olive oil and place in the oven.
8. Set the oven for about 7 minutes until toast are browned lightly. Remove from oven.
9. Divide the soup into bowls, cover with toast and splash with the cheese.
10. Place back to the oven at 350°F for about 10 minutes for cheese to bubble and browned lightly.
11. Serve immediately.

NUTRITIONAL INFORMATION

Calories: 468| Fat: 13g| Carbs: 65g| Protein: 21g| Sodium: 1897mg| Potassium: 729mg

INSTANT POT FRENCH ONION SOUP

This is a delicious and a tasty instant pot French onion soup that is a crowd pleaser as well as a time saver. It is a super easy Mediterranean lunch recipe requiring only a few ingredients and a few minutes to cook.

TIME: 25 MINUTES | **SERVINGS:** 6

INGREDIENTS

Veggies: 2 pounds peeled and sliced yellow onions, 3 minced garlic cloves

1 tbsp brown sugar

4 tbsp unsalted butter

3 tbsp flour

8 cups beef broth (college inn)

2 tbsp balsamic vinegar

For serving: 6 toasted baguette slices, 2 cups grated gruyere

METHOD

1. Place butter, onions, and sugar in an instant pot and sauté for about 20 minutes until onions are caramelized and golden brown.
2. Add garlic and flour stirring for flour to be cooked through.
3. Add vinegar and beef broth then seal the pot and cook for about 5 minutes under high pressure. Release pressure naturally.
4. Preheat the broiler then move the oven rack to the top position.
5. Divide the broth among 6 ovenproof bowls, top with a toast slice and splash with cheese generously.
6. Place the ovenproof bowls on a rimmed baking sheet.
7. Broil until cheese gets browned in spots and melts.
8. Serve and enjoy.

INSTANT POT GREEK LEMON CHICKEN SOUP

This is a light instant pot Greek lemon chicken soup that is refreshing. It is a perfect meal for Sunday supper with your family.

TIME: 33 MINUTES | **SERVINGS: 4**

INGREDIENTS

2 tbsp olive oil

2 chicken breasts (large and cubed to bite-size chunks)

Veggies: 1 medium finely diced onion, 4 minced garlic cloves, 2 large diced celery stalks, 1 bay leaf, fresh parsley(to garnish)

Spices: zest of one lemon, $\frac{1}{2}$ tbsp salt, $\frac{1}{4}$ tbsp black pepper (fresh cracked), pepper and salt to taste

Liquids: 4 cups chicken broth, juice of one lemon

1 large egg

METHOD

1. Turn instant pot to sauté mode and let it become hot.
2. Add 1 tbsp olive oil followed by the chicken and sauté until browned. Set aside.
3. Add 1 tbsp olive oil, onions, celery, and sauté for about 2 minutes.
4. Add garlic and sauté for another 1 minute.
5. Place the chicken back; add broth, pepper, lemon zest, salt, and bay leaf. Turn off sauté mode.
6. Seal the pot and cook for about 20 minutes under manual setting then allow pressure to release naturally for about 3 minutes. Quick release the rest.
7. Whisk egg in a bowl (medium); add lemon juice and whisk again to combine.
8. Add $\frac{1}{2}$ cup broth and lemon mixture and mix continuously.
9. Transfer the egg mixture to the soup stirring constantly.
10. Top with parsley.
11. Serve immediately.

NUTRITIONAL INFORMATION

Calories: 201 | Fat: 10.75g | Carbs: 4.75g | Protein: 17.8g | Sodium: 1087mg | Potassium: 270.75mg

Chapter 5: Red Meat Recipes

INSTANT POT BEEF GYROS WITH TZATZIKI SAUCE

This is an instant pot beef recipe that is tender and is ready in less than 70 minutes. It is a juicy and healthy Mediterranean dish that contains beef. Beef is a very good source of carnosine, which helps in the reduction of fatigue thus improve performance in exercise.

TIME: 1 HOUR | **SERVINGS:** 6

INGREDIENTS

$1\frac{1}{2}$ Lbs. roast beef cross rib (thinly sliced

Liquid: 2 tbsp olive oil, $\frac{1}{3}$ cup beef broth, 2 tbsp lemon juice (fresh)

Spices: 2 tbsp garlic powder, 1 tbsp salt, $\frac{1}{2}$ tbsp pepper, 2 tbsp oregano, 1 large thinly sliced onion

Veggies: lettuce, tomatoes

Soft pita bread

FOR TZATZIKI SAUCE

1 cup Greek yogurt (plain), 1 cup cucumber (diced, shredded and seeded), 1 tbsp dried dill, $\frac{1}{4}$ tbsp salt, 1 minced garlic clove

METHOD

1. Add beef, olive oil, onion, garlic powder, pepper, $\frac{3}{4}$ tbsp salt, beef broth and lemon juice in an instant pot.
2. Seal the pot and cook for about 25 minutes under manual high pressure then release pressure naturally for about 15 minutes. Unseal the pot and stir seasoning with pepper and salt.
3. **To make tzatziki sauce:** place all ingredients for tzatziki sauce in a bowl then stir until combined and creamy. Season with pepper and salt.
4. Serve the beef with the sauce, lettuce, tomatoes, onions, and feta.
5. Enjoy

INSTANT POT MISSISSIPI ROAST GYROS

This is a Mediterranean instant pot dish that everyone will love. Topping with sour cream and Monterey jack cheese makes it more delicious and perfect for lunch.

TIME: 1 HOUR 15 MINUTES | **SERVINGS:** 8

INGREDIENTS

2 pounds cross rib roast

Liquid: $\frac{1}{2}$ Cup water, $\frac{1}{2}$ Cup pepperoncini juice, $\frac{1}{4}$ Cup divided butter, $\frac{1}{2}$ Cup sour cream

Spices: 1 tbsp better than bouillon beef base, 1 tbsp salt (kosher), 1 tbsp onion powder, 1 tbsp garlic powder, $\frac{1}{4}$ Tbsp black pepper, $\frac{1}{4}$ Tbsp thyme (dried)

Veggies: 5 pepperoncini's,

8 pitas

$\frac{1}{2}$ Cup Monterey Jack cheese (grated)

METHOD

1. Heat your instant pot under sauté function.
2. Meanwhile, cut the rib roast half lengthwise then add 2 tbsp butter to the pot to melt.
3. Add the roast pieces and cook for about 5 minutes on each side until browned. Transfer to a plate.
4. Deglaze the instant pot using water then add beef base and let it dissolve in water. Add pepperoncini juice.
5. Place the roast pieces back to the pot then snuggle pepperoncinis round the roast pieces.
6. Add another 2 tbsp of butter then splash the roast pieces with onion powder, salt, thyme, garlic powder, and black pepper.
7. Seal the pot and cook for about 60 minutes under manual high pressure then release pressure naturally for about 20 minutes. Quick release remaining pressure.
8. Place the roast pieces on a cutting board and shred. Place back to the pot and stir with the juices.
9. Divide the meat among 8 warmed pitas then top with cheese and sour cream.
10. Roll up, serve and enjoy!

INSTANT POT GREEK BEEF STEW

This is a hearty and rich instant pot dish that is easy to prepare for dinner. It is a delicious Mediterranean Greek beef stew perfect for cold weather. Make it in during the winter season, and everyone will enjoy.

TIME: 55 MINUTES | **SERVINGS:** 4

INGREDIENTS

$1\frac{1}{2}$ Lbs. stew beef (1-inch cubes cut)

$\frac{1}{4}$ Cup butter

Veggies: 8 onions (small), 8 potatoes (small), 2-3 sliced carrots

Spices: 1 tbsp cinnamon, $\frac{3}{4}$ Cup tomato paste, salt, and pepper to taste

METHOD

1. Turn pot to sauté mode then add butter and beef. Cook for about 5 minutes until brown and transfer to a bowl.
2. Add onions with liquid (small amount) and sauté for about 5 minutes. Turn off sauté mode.
3. Place the beef back to the pot along with cinnamon, potatoes, tomato paste, and carrots.
4. Add about 3 cups water enough to cover the ingredients.
5. Seal the pot, set to the pressure cooker and cook for about 35 minutes under high pressure.
6. Release pressure naturally for about 10 minutes then quick release the remaining pressure.
7. Serve along warm, nice loaf bread.

NUTRITIONAL INFORMATION

Calories: 479 | Fat: 20g | Carbs: 31g | Protein: 43g | Sodium: 618mg | Potassium: 1703mg

BEEF GYRO

This is an easy, delicious Mediterranean beef gyro perfect for a weeknight dinner. When prepared in an instant pot, the beef becomes very tender for everyone to enjoy.

TIME: 50 MINUTES | **SERVINGS:** 6

INGREDIENTS

2 lbs. beef roast ($\frac{1}{4}$ inch sliced)

Spices: 1 tbsp salt, 1 tbsp garlic powder, 1 tbsp oregano

Liquid: 2 tbsp lemon juice, $\frac{1}{2}$ cup beef broth

For tzatziki sauce: 1 cup Greek yogurt, 2 tbsp minced garlic, 1 tbsp red wine vinegar, 1 tbsp lemon juice, pepper, and salt

For toppings: diced tomatoes, diced cucumber, thinly sliced red onion, 6 pita bread

METHOD

1. Place the beef roast, spices, and the liquids in the instant pot and seal the pot.
2. Cook for about 30 minutes using meat/stew setting the release pressure naturally.
3. Prepare tzatziki sauce by combining all its ingredients.
4. Serve the beef with the sauce and top with the toppings.

NUTRITIONAL INFORMATION

Calories: 387 | Fat: 8g | Carbs: 33g | Protein: 41g | Sodium: 854mg | Potassium: 646mg

INSTANT POT GREEK LAMB BEEF GYROS

This is a Mediterranean recipe that you will not have enough of. It is easy, healthy and a delicious instant pot dish perfectly awesome for dinner or lunch.

TIME: 45 MINUTES | **SERVINGS:** 4

INGREDIENTS

2 lb. ground lamb

Spices: 2 tbsp ground marjoram, 2 tbsp dried oregano, 2 tbsp dried rosemary, $\frac{1}{4}$ tbsp black pepper (freshly ground), 2 tbsp kosher salt,

Veggies: 5-oz brown onion (small), 8 fresh garlic cloves

To serve: 2 cups tzatziki sauce, feta cheese, 4 Greek pitas, brown onion, cucumber, lettuce, tomatoes (fresh and chopped)

METHOD

1. Chop the onion well using a food processor then use a paper towel to squeeze out the liquid from the onion.
2. Place the dry onion back to the processor and add garlic, rosemary, marjoram, oregano, pepper, and salt. Process until garlic gets minced.
3. Add ground lamb and process until combined well.
4. Place the meat mixture on loaf pan and press until compact and very tight. Cover with a tin foil tightly then make vent holes on the foil.
5. Place 1 $\frac{1}{2}$ cups water in the instant pot with a trivet inside then place the loaf pan on the trivet.
6. Seal the pot and set to pressure cooking.
7. Cook for about 15 minutes under manual high pressure then release pressure naturally.
8. Unseal the pot and remove the loaf pan. Separate the gyro meat from the pan and slice thin.
9. Serve with the serving ingredients.

PEPPERONCINI ITALIAN BEEF

This is a spicy and a delicious pepperoncini roast that is great and can be served as a sandwich on the hoagie roll. It is an instant pot Italian beef with only 4 ingredients perfect for busy weeknights.

TIME: 1 HOUR 5 MINUTES | **SERVINGS:** 6

INGREDIENTS

3 lbs of beef roast

16 oz can pepperoncini peppers (with the liquid)

1 packet Italian salad dressing mix (dry)

1 packet gravy mix (brown)

METHOD

1. Place everything in the instant pot and seal the pot.
2. Cook for about 1 hour under manual high pressure then release pressure naturally.
3. Let it rest for about 5 minutes and shred the beef chunks to allow pepper and juice to mix in with the beef.
4. Serve and enjoy!

NUTRITIONAL INFORMATION

Calories: 293 | Fat: 8g | Carbs: 4g | Protein: 50g | Sodium: 3425mg | Potassium: 828mg

EASY INSTANT POT ITALIAN BEEF

This Italian beef is full of flavors and spices enough to be a crowd pleaser. It is super easy when prepared in the instant pot and is great for holidays or even birthday parties.

TIME: 1 HOUR 10 MINUTES | **SERVINGS:** 8

INGREDIENTS

$2\frac{1}{2}$ - $3\frac{1}{2}$ lb. chunk beef roast (2-inches thick)

Spices: 1 tbsp Italian seasoning, 1 tbsp black pepper, 2 tbsp kosher salt, 1 tbsp Worcestershire sauce

Veggies: 1 jar pepperoncini peppers (sliced), 3 smashed garlic cloves, 1 roughly chopped onion, 1 roughly chopped bell pepper

Ciabatta or hoagie roll

METHOD

1. Heat your instant pot under sauté mode. Meanwhile, season the beef roast with the spices.
2. Splash olive oil to the pot and cook the beef roast to browning on both sides.
3. Add bell peppers, onions and garlic cloves on the roast top then dump the pepperoncini peppers and the Worcestershire sauce.
4. Seal the pot and cook for about 55 minutes under manual high pressure. Release pressure naturally.
5. Unseal the pot then remove the beef roast and shred. Place the beef roast back to the pot.
6. Serve on the buttered and toasted rolls

INSTANT POT ITALIAN BEEF

This is the easiest Mediterranean recipe you will ever make. It is a recipe that all ingredients are put in the instant and left to cook. That's it.

TIME: 1 HOUR 15 MINUTES | **SERVINGS: 8**

INGREDIENTS

4-5 lb. beef chuck roast

Spices: 1 packet Italian dressing mix (dry), 1 cup beef broth

16-ounce jar pepperoncini rings

Provolone cheese slices

Hoagie buns

METHOD

1. Place the roast in the instant pot and top with beef broth, Italian dressing mix, and 1 cup pepperoncini rings.
2. Cook for about 1 hour under high pressure then release pressure naturally for about 10 minutes. Quick release the rest.
3. Preheat the boiler. In the meantime, shred the beef roast.
4. Place the bottoms of hoagie rolls on a baking sheet.
5. Heap the beef roast on the hoagie buns, few tbsp of broth over the beef and top with the cheese.
6. Broil for the cheese to melt.
7. Top with pepperoncini rings remainder and hoagie bun top.
8. Serve and enjoy.

INSTANT POT EASY ITALIAN BEEF

This is a Mediterranean recipe that you will absolutely love as it is easy, full of flavors and the meat is so tender. It is an instant pot dish perfect for summer days.

TIME: 1 HOUR 10 MINUTES | **SERVINGS:** 8

INGREDIENTS

5-6 lbs. chuck roast

1 tbsp canola oil

7 oz. Italian dressing seasoning mix

Veggies: 16 oz. Pepperoncini peppers (sliced), $\frac{1}{2}$ thinly sliced yellow onion

1 cup water

METHOD

1. Set your instant to sauté mode then add canola oil.
2. Brown the roast, once hot, for about 6 minutes on each side.
3. Add onions, water, Italian seasoning mix, half of pepperoncini pepper and $\frac{1}{4}$ cup pepperoncini brine.
4. Seal the pot and cook for about 55 minutes under manual high pressure then release pressure naturally.
5. Unseal the pot and shred the roast with forks.
6. Add the pepperoncini peppers remainder which has been drained.
7. Serve and enjoy!

NUTRITIONAL INFORMATION

Calories: 651 | Fat: 41g | Carbs: 4g | Protein: 66g | Sodium: 544mg | Potassium: 1284mg

INSTANT POT SWEET AND SPICY MEATBALLS

This is a fabulous instant pot dish that is super delicious. Beef is a very good source of carnosine, which helps to reduce fatigue, thereby improving performance in exercise. The healthy profile makes this Mediterranean recipe perfect for the family dish.

TIME: 55 MINUTES | **SERVINGS:** 4

INGREDIENTS

1 pound ground beef (chopped)

$\frac{1}{4}$ Cup bread crumbs

1 egg

Spices: 2 tbsp ketchup, 1 cup marinara, 1 cup tzatziki sauce

2 tbsp water

METHOD

1. Mix beef, ketchup, bread crumbs, egg, pepper, and salt then shape the mixture into balls.
2. Place the balls in the instant pot at the bottom.
3. In the meantime, mix marinara and the tzatziki sauce then pour over the meatballs.
4. Seal the pot and turn on to meat/stew mode. Cook for about 45 minutes under manual high pressure then release pressure naturally.
5. Serve over rice.
6. Enjoy!

Chapter 6: Poultry Recipes
INSTANT POT TURKEY STUFFED SWEET POTATOES

This is a perfect instant pot turkey recipe that takes only 30 minutes to prepare. It is a healthy and delicious Mediterranean meal that everyone will absolutely love.

TIME: 30 MINUTES | **SERVINGS:** 4

INGREDIENTS

$1\frac{1}{2}$ cup water

2 sweet potatoes

75 lb. Italian turkey

2 tbsp avocado oil

Optional: 4 cups spinach

METHOD

1. Pour water in the instant pot with a rack inside then place the potatoes on the rack.
2. Use the pack instructions to cook the sweet potatoes until done then safely release pressure naturally.
3. Transfer the sweet potatoes to a bowl and cut to half and drain the pot.
4. Set instant pot to sauté settings then add oil and onions. Sauté until onions become tender and translucent.
5. Add turkey, and sauté under low setting until cooked through.
6. Optional: add the spinach and sauté to wilting.
7. Mush the sweet potatoes with a fork to the center down. Make sure you fill the sweet potatoes with the meat filling.
8. Serve.

NUTRITIONAL INFORMATION

Calories: 458 | Fat: 18g | Carbs: 42g | Protein: 32g

INSTANT POT CHICKEN THIGHS WITH SUN-DRIED TOMATOES AND ARTICHOKES

This is the easiest Mediterranean recipe perfect for Sunday morning. It is an instant pot recipe that everyone will absolutely love and will amazingly melt your mouth with flavor and texture.

TIME: 5 HOURS 55 MINUTES | **SERVINGS:** 6

INGREDIENTS

6 chicken thighs (boneless)

Spices: $\frac{1}{2}$ Tbsp oregano (dried), 4 minced garlic cloves, 3 tbsp chopped parsley (fresh)

$14\frac{3}{4}$ ounces artichoke hearts (drained, Cara mia) + $\frac{1}{3}$ cup artichoke hearts liquid

$3\frac{1}{2}$ ounces sun-dried tomatoes (julienne)

Pepper and salt to taste

METHOD

1. Set your instant pot to slow cooker and spray inside with cooking spray.
2. Meanwhile, season the chicken with pepper, salt and oregano, and place to the pot.
3. Place the tomatoes and artichoke over the chicken then splash with garlic.
4. Pour $\frac{1}{3}$ cup of the artichoke hearts liquid over.
5. Cook on slow cooker mode for about 4 $\frac{1}{2}$ hours under high pressure. Release pressure naturally.
6. Transfer to plates and splash with parsley.
7. Enjoy.

NUTRITIONAL INFORMATION

Calories: 169 | Fat: 12g | Carbs: 1g | Protein: 12g | Sodium: 60mg | Potassium: 173mg

INSTANT POT MEDITERRANEAN TURKEY CUTLETS

This is a delicious Mediterranean dish that is served with tomato ketchup. Turkey contains niacin and B6 which are essential for the production of energy in the body.

TIME: 20 MINUTES | **SERVINGS:** 6

INGREDIENTS

2 pounds turkey cutlets

4 tbsp olive oil

2 tbsp turmeric powder

2 tbsp Greek seasoning

1 cup flour (all-purpose)

METHOD

1. Mix flour and the cutlets and set aside to marinade for about 10 minutes.
2. Pour olive oil to the instant pot then add half the cutlets to the pot.
3. Cook for about 5 minutes under manual high pressure then release pressure naturally.
4. Transfer to a plate.
5. Repeat for the other of the cutlets.
6. Serve and enjoy.

INSTANT POT MEDITERRANEAN CHICKEN

This is an easy and delicious Mediterranean instant pot dish to have for dinner. It is a healthy and perfect recipe for bodybuilders since chicken is rich in protein which contributes to growth and development of muscles.

TIME: 20 MINUTES | **SERVINGS:** 6

INGREDIENTS

2 lb. chicken tenders (frozen)

Veggies: 1 chopped onion, $\frac{1}{2}$ Chopped green pepper

Spices: 4 crushed garlic cloves, 1 can black olives (sliced)

$\frac{1}{2}$ Cup crumbled feta

2 cans (15-oz) stewed tomatoes

METHOD

1. Put all ingredients in an instant pot apart from feta.
2. Cook for about 14 minutes under high pressure then quick-release pressure.
3. Serve with a grain of your choice and top with crumbled feta.
4. Enjoy.

INSTANT POT MEDITERRANEAN CHICKEN AND RICE BOWL

This is a super easy Mediterranean chicken dish to have for dinner. It is a perfect instant pot dish bowl with amazing flavors, and it takes only 30 minutes to be ready.

TIME: 30 MINUTES | **SERVINGS:** 6

INGREDIENTS

$1\frac{1}{2}$ lb. frozen chicken breasts (boneless and skinless)

Spices: 2 cups chopped bell peppers, $1\frac{1}{2}$ cup chicken broth (low-sodium), One-lemon juice

2 cups artichoke hearts (soaked and drained)

1 cup brown rice

2 tbsp olive oil

Toppings: $\frac{1}{2}$ cup toasted pine nuts and finely chopped basil

METHOD

1. Turn instant pot to sauté mode then heat oil and add bell pepper and artichoke hearts.
2. Sauté for about 5 minutes until browned a little then turn off the pot.
3. Add chicken breasts, pepper, salt, and lemon juice then pour the rice over them. Add chicken broth.
4. Seal the pot and cook over manual settings for about 20 minutes then release the pressure naturally for about 10 minutes. Quick release any pressure remaining.
5. Unseal the pot and shred the chicken with a fork then mix the ingredients now.
6. Transfer to a bowl and pour the toppings over.
7. Serve.

NUTRITIONAL INFORMATION

Calories: 310| Carbs: 32g| Protein: 6g| Fat: 16g| Sodium: 274mg| Potassium: 307mg| Fiber: 3g

INSTANT POT SWEET AND SPICY MEATBALLS

This is an easy instant pot turkey meatballs that are flavorful and delicious. It is a healthy Mediterranean recipe since turkey is rich in protein, selenium, and potassium which help in strengthening the immune system.

TIME: 55 MINUTES | **SERVINGS:** 4

INGREDIENTS

1 pound turkey (chopped)

$\frac{1}{4}$ Cup bread crumbs

1 egg

Spices: 2 tbsp ketchup, 1 cup marinara, 1 cup duck sauce (spicy)

Pepper and salt to taste

METHOD

1. Mix chopped turkey, egg, bread crumbs, ketchup, pepper and salt with 2 tbsp water then shape into balls.
2. Place in the bottom of your instant pot. Meanwhile, mix duck sauce and marinara.
3. Pour the marinara mixture over the meatballs then seal the pot and turn instant pot to meat.
4. Cook for about 45 minutes then release pressure naturally.
5. Serve with rice.

INSTANT POT CHICKEN AND SWEET POTATOES

This is sweet, easy, and delicious Mediterranean instant pot dish to enjoy with your family. It is a healthy recipe since sweet potatoes are a good source of antioxidants (beta-carotene and anthocyanins) which improve eye health.

TIME: 45 minutes | **SERVINGS:** 8

INGREDIENTS

16 ounces sweet potatoes (diced)

1 pound chicken breasts

Spices: 3 tbsp buffalo sauce, Garlic powder, onion (each, $\frac{1}{2}$ tbsp)

3 tbsp butter

1 onion (diced)

METHOD

1. Turn your instant pot to sauté mode and place in onions and 1 tbsp butter.
2. Sauté until brown then add chicken, sweet potatoes, 2 tbsp butter, and buffalo sauce.
3. Seal the pot and set to poultry mode. (If using frozen chicken, cook the chicken for about 30 minutes under manual function).
4. Quick release pressure and serve.

DUCK AND VEGGIES

This is a delicious Mediterranean instant pot recipe that is very easy to prepare. Duck meat is a rich source of copper and other minerals which help maintain a strong and stable mental health as well as physical health.

TIME: 30 MINUTES | **SERVINGS:** 8

INGREDIENTS

1 duck (medium-size)

2 carrots (cut to pieces)

1 cucumber (cut to pieces)

2 tbsp wine + 1tbsp cooking wine

1 ginger (small and cut to pieces)

METHOD

1. Place all ingredients with 2 cups water in the instant pot. Season with salt to taste.
2. Seal the pot and Turn the pot to meat-stew mode. Cook on manual function for about 20 minutes then release pressure for about 10 minutes.
3. Serve and enjoy.

MEDITERRANEAN WHOLE CHICKEN

This is a perfect instant pot chicken for dinner. The Mediterranean recipe is delicious and healthy since chicken is rich in protein which contributes to growth and development of muscles.

TIME: 18 MINUTES | **SERVINGS:** 4

INGREDIENTS

1 whole chicken

1 tbsp coconut oil

1 cup water

Pepper and salt to taste

Mediterranean Seasoning of your choice

METHOD

1. Pour water in your instant pot with a steam rack inside. Meanwhile, preheat oil in a skillet (large).
2. Flavor the chicken with favorite Mediterranean seasoning then sear on the skillet for about 1 minute on each side.
3. Place flavored chicken on the steam rack, seal the pot and cook under high pressure for about 12 minutes.
4. Release pressure naturally and unseal the pot.
5. Serve warm.

INSTANT POT MEDITERRANEAN PASTA CHICKEN

This is a fast and easy instant pot Mediterranean recipe perfect for a busy weeknight dinner. Chicken is rich in protein which contributes to growth and development of muscles making this a healthy dish

TIME: 45 MINUTES | **SERVINGS:** 4

INGREDIENTS

3 chicken breasts (large, skinless and boneless)

Spices: 1 cup chicken broth, 2 cups marinara sauce

Veggies: 1 (14.5 Oz) tomatoes (diced and with juice) + $\frac{1}{2}$ cup sun-dried, 1 tbsp chopped peppers (roasted and jarred), $\frac{1}{2}$ Cup kalamata olives

9 Oz Penne pasta

METHOD

1. Place everything apart from the pasta in the instant pot and seal the pot.
2. Cook for about 12 minutes under manual setting the release pressure naturally. Unseal the pot.
3. Now add the pasta and seal the pot again. Cook for another 5 minutes under manual setting.
4. Release pressure naturally for about 5 minutes and quick release the rest.
5. Serve and enjoy

NUTRITIONAL INFORMATION

Calories: 433 | Fat: 8g | Carbs: 40g | Protein: 47g

Chapter 7: Fish and Seafood

MEDITERRANEAN INSTANT POT FROZEN SALMON

Are you a seafood lover? This Mediterranean instant pot frozen pot is ready without being thawed and stays moist and warm. Add toppings such as sweet barbeque sauce, seasoned salt, butter and pesto sauce for flavor.

TIME: 10 MINUTES | **SERVINGS:** 2

INGREDIENTS

$\frac{1}{4}$ Cup lemon juice

Cooking spray

Salt and pepper to taste

2 salmon fillets (frozen)

Salad dressing of choice

METHOD

1. Pour lemon juice and a cup of cold water in your instant pot. Place the steamer rack in place and spray cooking spray.
2. Place the salmon on the steamer skin side facing down. Lid the instant pot then close the vent.
3. Set time for four minutes at the steam function. When time is done release pressure.
4. Season with pepper and salt.
5. Serve with your favorite salad.

NUTRITIONAL INFORMATION

Cal: 172 | Fat: 6.7g | Carbs: 2.6g | Fiber: 0.1g | Protein: 24.6g | Sugar: 1g

INSTANT POT SALMON

Cooking salmon in your instant pot is the easiest and quickest way to enjoy seafood dish. This salmon dish will be on your table within twenty minutes. It's delicious and worth a shot when on vacation at the beach.

TIME: 20 MINUTES | **SERVING:** 4

INGREDIENTS

1 cup water

1 lb. Alaskan salmon (wild caught and frozen)

Salt and pepper

METHOD

1. Pour water in the instant pot and place the metal trivet in place.
2. Place the fillets on the trivet in a single layer then sprinkle salt and pepper.
3. Lid the instant pot and set the valve to seal. Set time for five minutes at high pressure.
4. Quick release pressure and remove the fillet from the instant pot.
5. Serve with side dish of your choice and salad dressing

NUTRITIONAL INFORMATION

Cal: 172| Fat: 6.7g| Carbs: 2.6g| Fiber: 0.1g| Protein: 24.6g| Sugar: 1g

INSTANT POT SALMON WITH ROSEMARY

This is a delicious, healthy, and simple instant pot Mediterranean salmon with rosemary. This salmon is spiced up by the fresh rosemary sprig making it finger-licking sweet. The dish is worth a repeat dinner.

TIME: 6 MINUTES | **SERVING:** 4

INGREDIENTS

1 lb. salmon

1 cup water

2 sprigs rosemary

1 tbsp mustard powder

Salt and pepper to taste

METHOD

1. Pour water in your instant pot then place the steaming rack in place.
2. Place the salmon, or the rack then sprinkle rosemary followed by mustard powder and salt to taste.
3. Set time for five minutes at high pressure. When time is done release pressure naturally and serve when hot.

NUTRITIONAL INFORMATION

Cal: 88 | Fat: 12g | Carbs: 4.3g | Fiber: 2g | Protein: 32g | Sugar: 1.8g

MEDITERRANEAN STYLE INSTANT POT COD

This is a super easy instant pot cod that is delicious and perfect for seafood lovers. Make this cod for dinner for your family member and friends and serve it with your favorite sauce.

TIME: 15 MINUTES | **SERVING:** 6

INGREDIENTS

3 tbsp butter

6 pieces of cod

1 onion (sliced)

Spices: Salt and pepper to taste, 1 tbsp oregano

24 oz. can tomatoes (diced)

METHOD

1. Put on the sauté function on your instant pot. Melt the butter and add all other ingredients with lime juice and salt to taste to the instant pot except the fresh cod.
2. Stir to combine and cook for ten minutes.
3. Arrange the fish in the sauce then carefully cover each piece with the sauce. Lid and set valve to sealing. Set time for five minutes at high pressure. When time is done release pressure quickly and serve when hot with the sauce.
4. Enjoy.

CLEAN EATING MEDITERRANEAN ROSEMARY SALMON

What more can you ask for on top of this healthy, very delicious Mediterranean salmon, which is ready in a few minutes. Make this instant salmon for your family and friends for a surprise dinner.

TIME: 20 MINUTES | **SERVING:** 3

INGREDIENTS

1lb, salmon

10 oz. asparagus (fresh)

1 sprig rosemary

½ Cup cherry tomatoes (halved)

Salt and pepper to taste

METHOD

1. Pour a cup of water in your instant pot then place a wire rack in place.
2. Layer the salmon on the wire followed by asparagus and then the rosemary.
3. Set time for three minutes. When time is done release pressure, then remove the salmon from the instant pot.
4. Transfer the salmon to a plate and disposing the rosemary sprig. Add halved cherry tomatoes, one tbsp olive oil and salt, and pepper.
5. Sprinkle lemon juice if you desire.
6. Serve and enjoy.

NUTRITIONAL INFORMATION

Cal: 282 | Fat: 14g | Carbs: 5g | Fiber: 2g | Protein: 32g | Sugar: 2g

INSTANT POT MEDITERRANEAN FRESH COD

This is the great tasting classic seafood dish made from your home. This cod is juicy and fall off the bone tender. Serve this cod with garlic/mayonnaise to make it taste amazingly delicious.

TIME: 25 MINUTES | **SERVINGS:** 12

INGREDIENTS

12 Pieces cod (fresh or frozen)

Spices: 2 tbsp lemon juice, 2tbsp oregano, 28 oz. tomatoes (canned diced)

6 tbsp butter

Salt and pepper to taste

METHOD

1. Add all the ingredients in your instant pot except the cod then put on the sauté function.
2. Sauté for ten minutes then stir.
3. Add fish in the instant pot and ensure all fish is covered. Lid and set time for three minutes on high pressure.
4. When time is done release pressure naturally. Open the instant pot and remove the cod from the instant pot.
5. Serve and enjoy when hot.

INSTANT POT COD AND PEAS WITH SOUR CREAM

Are you on vacation at a beach and wondering what to prepare for dinner? Just grab your instant pot and prepare this cod in minutes. It is a simple and delicious seafood dish that is low in carbohydrate and low in calories.

TIME: 10 MINUTES | **SERVING:** 2

INGREDIENTS

4 cod fillets

Spices: 1 tbsp parsley (fresh), 1 garlic clove (chopped)

$\frac{1}{2}$ Lb. peas (frozen)

$\frac{1}{2}$ tbsp paprika

1 cup sour cream

METHOD

1. Place the steamer trivet in place in the instant pot and pour a cup of water in the instant pot.
2. Place the cod fillets on the trivet.
3. Lid the instant pot and set time for two minutes at high pressure. When time is done release pressure quickly.
4. Add peas in the steamer and cook for two more minutes under high pressure.
5. Meanwhile, add all other ingredients in your food processor and blend until smooth.
6. Pour the cream in a serving bowl then add the cod and peas. Serve and enjoy.

INSTANT POT DELICIOUS LOBSTER

This is an awesomely sweet lobster, rich in flavors and sweet aroma. It's dinner ready twenty-five minutes. Surprise your family members or friends with this insanely delicious and addictive dish.

TIME: 25 MINUTES | **SERVINGS:** 6

INGREDIENTS

1 tbsp bay seasoning (old)

2 lb. lobster tails (fresh)

Spices: 2 tbsp lemon juice (fresh), $\frac{1}{2}$ Cup mayonnaise

1 scallion (chopped)

2 tbsp butter (unsalted)

METHOD

1. Place the steamer trivet in place in your instant pot then add a cup of water and a pinch bay seasoning.
2. Arrange the lobster on the trivet (shell side down).
3. Drizzle half the lemon juice then lid the instant pot and set time for three minutes at high pressure.
4. Release pressure quickly then transfer the lobster to an ice bath bowl to rest.
5. Use kitchen shears to cut down to Centre, the underbelly of the lobster tail.
6. Remove meat chopping it into chunks.
7. In a large serving bowl add the lobster, chopped scallions, mayonnaise, unsalted butter, remaining seasoning, and lemon juice then mix.
8. Put in a fridge for fifteen minutes before serving.

INSTANT POT SWEET AND SOUR FISH

This simple, traditional, excellently delicious instant pot Mediterranean sour fish requires very few ingredients and just twenty minutes to be ready. It's loved by kids and will definitely be your family favorite.

TIME: 20 MINUTES | **SERVINGS: 6**

INGREDIENTS

1 tbsp olive oil

1 tbsp sugar

Spices: 2 tbsp soy sauce, 2 tbsp vinegar

2 lb. fish chunks

Mediterranean salad for serving

METHOD

1. Put olive oil and fish in your instant pot .put the sauté function on.
2. Cook for three minutes then add all the other ingredients.
3. Set time for six minutes at high pressure. When time is done release pressure naturally and remove the fish.
4. Serve and enjoy with salad

MEDITERRANEAN INSTANT POT STEAMED CRAB LEGS

This is a perfect and delicious dinner choice you can ever make for your loved ones. It's easy, light and very healthy when served with salads, and lemon juice. These crab legs with salad will highly compliment your Mediterranean diet.

TIME: 7 MINUTES | **SERVING:** 4

INGREDIENTS

2 lb. crab legs (frozen)

4 tbsp butter

Lemon juice to taste and for serving

Salad of choice

METHOD

1. Place the trivet in place on the instant pot then place the crab legs on the trivet.
2. Add three-quarter of water in the instant pot then lid the instant pot. Set time for two minutes on high pressure.
3. Quickly release pressure and remove the crab legs from the instant pot.
4. Mix butter and lemon juice then drizzle over crab legs.
5. Serve with salad, lemon wedges and a salad of choice.

Chapter 8: Vegan and Vegetarian Recipes

INSTANT POT BLACK EYED PEAS

This instant pot black peas is an awesome lunch or dinner that will keep your family full until the next meal. It's rich in flavors and will leave your taste buds thanking you and yearning for more.

TIME: 30 minutes | **Servings:** 4

INGREDIENTS

2 cups black-eyed peas (dried)

1 cup Olive oil

Spices: 1 cup parsley (stem removed and chopped), 1 cup dill (fresh, stem removed and chopped), 2 slices oranges (fresh), 2 bay leaves, 2 tbsp tomato paste, salt and pepper to taste

Veggies: 4 green onions (thinly sliced), 2 carrots (sliced),

METHOD

1. Clean the dill thoroughly with water removing stones.
2. Add all the ingredients in the instant pot and stir well to combine.
3. Lid the instant pot and set the vent to sealing.
4. Set time for twenty-five minutes. When the time has elapsed release pressure naturally.
5. Serve and enjoy the black eyed peas.

INSTANT POT FASOLAKIA (GREEN BEANS AND POTATOES IN OLIVE OIL)

Are you a Mediterranean diet lover? Beans are really a big deal in the Mediterranean diet. These green beans and potatoes are perfectly delicious and surprisingly ready in fifteen minutes in your instant pot.

TIME: 30 MINUTES | **SERVING:** 4

INGREDIENTS

15 oz. tomatoes (diced)

$\frac{1}{2}$ Cup virgin olive oil

Veggies: 1 zucchini (quartered), 2 potatoes (quartered), 1 lb. green beans (fresh)

Spices: 1 bunch dill, 1 tbs dried oregano, $\frac{1}{2}$ bunch parsley (chopped)

METHOD

1. Turn on the sauté function on your instant pot.
2. Pour tomatoes, a cup of water and olive oil. Add the rest of the ingredients and stir through.
3. Lid the instant pot and set the valve to seal. Set time for fifteen minutes.
4. When the time has elapsed release pressure. Remove the Fasolakia from the instant pot. Serve and enjoy.

NUTRITIOUS VEGAN CABBAGE

This simple and nutritious vegan cabbage soup is perfect for the Mediterranean diet and for a detox. It takes thirty minutes in your instant pot to get this soup ready. This cabbage soup is insanely delicious and addictive.

TIME: 50 MINUTES | **SERVING:** 6

INGREDIENTS

Veggies: 3 cups green cabbage (coarsely chopped), 1 can tomatoes (diced), 3 carrots (chopped), 1 onion

$2\frac{1}{2}$ Cups vegetable broth

Spices: (2 garlic, 3 stalks celery (chopped), 2 tbsp vinegar (apple cider), 1 tbsp lemon juice, 2 tbsp sage (dried))

METHOD

1. Add all the ingredients in the instant pot. Lid and set time for fifteen minutes on high pressure.
2. Release pressure naturally then remove the lid. Remove the soup from the instant pot.
3. Serve and enjoy.

NUTRITIONAL INFORMATION

Cal: 67 | Fat: 0.4g | Carbs: 13.4g | Fiber: 3.8g | Protein: 2.3g | Sugar: 7g

INSTANT POT HORTA AND POTATOES

This instant pot Horta is quite popular in Mediterranean living. It's a Hit in most vegetarian homes. It's very easy to prepare, quick and amazingly sweet. Ensure you try it for your family, and they will love it.

TIME: 30 MINUTES | **SERVING:** 4

INGREDIENTS

2 heads of washed and chopped greens (spinach, Dandelion, kale, mustard green, Swiss chard)

6 potatoes (washed and cut in pieces)

1 cup virgin olive oil

1 lemon juice (reserve slices for serving)

10 garlic cloves (chopped)

METHOD

1. Put all the ingredients in the instant pot and lid setting the vent to sealing.
2. Set time for fifteen minutes. When time is done release pressure.
3. Let the potatoes rest for some time. Serve and enjoy with lemon slices.

INSTANT POT JACKFRUIT CURRY

This is a delicious main dish to prepare in your instant pot over the weeknight. It's easy to prepare and will blow away your family member's taste buds. Make sure to try this in your home.

TIME: 1 HOUR | **SERVING:** 2

INGREDIENTS

1 tbsp oil

Seeds: $\frac{1}{2}$ Cumin seeds, $\frac{1}{2}$ Mustard seeds, $\frac{1}{2}$ tbsp nigella seeds

Veggies: 1 onion (chopped), 2 tomatoes (purred)

20 oz. can green jackfruit (drained and rinsed)

Spices: 2 red chilies (dried), 2 bay leaves, 5 garlic cloves, ginger (chopped), 1 tbsp coriander powder, $\frac{1}{2}$ tbsp turmeric.

METHOD

1. Turn the instant pot to sauté mode. Add cumin seeds, mustard ten nigella seeds and allow them to sizzle.
2. Add red chilies and bay leaves and allow to cook for a few seconds.
3. Add chopped onion, garlic cloves, ginger and salt, and pepper to taste. Stir cook for five minutes.
4. Add other ingredients, and a cup of water then lid the instant pot. Set time for seven minutes on high pressure.
5. When the time has elapsed release pressure naturally, shred the jackfruit and serve.
6. Enjoy.

NUTRITIONAL INFORMATION

Cal: 369 | Fat: 3g | Carbs: 86g | Fiber: 6g | Protein: 4g | Sugar: 8g

INSTANT POT COLLARD GREENS WITH TOMATOES

Are you in search of the perfect side dish that will blow away your family or friends' taste buds and satisfy them? This plant-based collard greens with tomatoes are awesomely delicious and will surely satisfy friends and family.

TIME: 25 MINUTES | **SERVING:** 4

INGREDIENTS

1 white onion (diced)

3tbsp olive oil

3 garlic cloves (minced)

$\frac{1}{3}$ Cup tomatoes (sun-dried and chopped)

1 bunch collard greens (roughly cut and hard stems removed)

METHOD

1. Turn on the sauté function on your instant pot.
2. Add onions and olive oil to the instant pot and let cook for three minutes or until lightly browned.
3. Add the rest of ingredients one at a time while stirring.
4. Add salt and pepper to taste and a cup of water. Turn off the sauté function and set to manual. Set time for five minutes at high pressure.
5. When the time has elapsed, release pressure naturally.
6. Open the lid and drizzle a half lemon juice.
7. Serve and enjoy.

INSTANT POT ARTICHOKES WITH MEDITERRANEAN AIOLI

These instant pot artichokes are not only nutritious but also easy to make, delicious and insanely addictive. This is a paleo vegetarian dish each member of your family will really love and will ask for a repeat.

TIME: 15 MINUTES | **SERVING:** 3

INGREDIENTS

3 medium artichokes (stems cut off)

1 cup vegetable broth

Mediterranean aioli

METHOD

1. Place wire trivet in place in the instant pot then place the artichokes on the wire.
2. Pour vegetable broth over artichokes.
3. Lid the instant pot and put steam mode on. Set time for 10 minutes. When the time has elapsed allow pressure to release.
4. Remove the artichokes from the instant pot and reserve the remaining broth, about a quarter cup.
5. Half the artichokes and place them on serving bowls. Drizzle broth.
6. Serve with aioli and enjoy.

NUTRITIONAL INFORMATION

Cal: 30 | Fat: 0.1g | Carbs: 6.5g | Fiber: 3.5g | Protein: 2.1g | Sugar: 0.6g

INSTANT POT MILLET PILAF

This vegan millet pilaf is flavorful, healthy, and high in fiber. It is a delicious side dish studded with pistachios and dried apricots. It's easy to make and requires a few ingredients to prepare.

TIME: 30 MINUTES | **SERVING:** 4

INGREDIENTS

1 cup millet

$\frac{1}{4}$ Cup apricot and $\frac{1}{4}$ shelled pistachios (roughly chopped)

1 lemon juice and zest

$1\frac{1}{2}$ tbsp olive oil

$\frac{1}{2}$ Cup parsley (fresh)

METHOD

1. Pour one and three-quarter cup of water in your instant pot. Place the millet and lid the instant pot.
2. Set time for 10 minutes on high pressure. When the time has elapsed, release pressure naturally.
3. Remove the lid and add all other ingredients. Stir while adjusting the seasonings.
4. Serve and enjoy

NUTRITIONAL INFORMATION

Cal: 308 | Fat: 11g | Carbs: 46g | Fiber: 6g | Protein: 7g | Sugar: 5g

INSTANT POT STUFFED SWEET POTATOES

Are you sweet potatoes lover? Then these stuffed sweet potatoes are a must try. They are tasty, easy and ready in thirty minutes. These tender, sweet potatoes are rich in Mediterranean flavors, making them irresistibly sweet.

TIME: 35 MINUTES | **SERVING:** 2

INGREDIENTS

2 sweet potatoes (washed thoroughly)

1 cup chickpeas (cooked)

Olive oil

2 onions (cut)

Paprika

Toppings: (2 spring onions, 1 avocado (peeled and cut into half), cooked couscous, 1 lemon, 3 oz. feta cheese)

METHOD

1. Pour a cup and half of water in your instant pot then place steam rack in place.
2. Place the sweet potatoes on the rack. Set the valve to sealing and time for seventeen minutes under high pressure.
3. Meanwhile, roast the chickpeas on your pan with olive oil.
4. Add salt and pepper to taste then paprika. Stir until chickpeas are coated evenly.
5. Cook for a minute then put off the heat.
6. When the instant pot time elapses, release pressure naturally for five minutes. Let the sweet potatoes cool then remove them from the instant pot.
7. Cut the sweet potatoes lengthwise and use a fork to mash the inside creating a space for toppings.
8. Add the pre-prepared toppings then serve with feta cheese lemon wedges.

NUTRITIONAL INFORMATION

Cal: 776| Fat: 26g| Carbs: 116g| Fiber: 25g| Protein: 23g| Sugar: 20g

INSTANT POT COUSCOUS AND VEGETABLE MEDLEY

This is an awesomely delicious couscous cooked with your favorite vegetables in your instant pot. It can be served as a side dish, salad, and snack or in the morning for breakfast.

TIME: 25 MINUTES | **SERVINGS:** 3

INGREDIENTS

1 tbsp olive oil

Veggies: $\frac{1}{2}$ Onion (chopped), 1 cup carrot (grated), 1 red bell pepper (chopped)

1 $\frac{3}{4}$ cup couscous Israeli

Spices: Garam masala, cilantro, lemon juice, 2 bays leafs

METHOD

1. Put on sauté function on your instant pot then add olive oil.
2. Add bay leaves followed by chopped onions the sauté for two minutes.
3. Add pepper and carrots then continue to sauté for one more minute.
4. Stir in couscous, Garam masala, salt to taste and a cup and three-quarter of water.
5. Switch the sauté function to manual and set for two minutes. When the time has elapsed naturally release pressure for ten minutes.
6. Fluff the couscous then mix in lemon juice and garnish with cilantro.
7. Remove from instant pot and serve when hot

NUTRITIONAL INFORMATION

Cal: 460 | Fat: 5g | Carbs: 86g | Fiber: 7g | Protein: 13g | Sugar: 4g

Chapter 9: Snacks and Dessert Recipes

NATILLAS DE LECHE (SPANISH CUSTARD)

This is a delicious meal rich in yellow color, creamy, thick and above all nutritious. The flavors in this Spanish custard will blow you away and won't regret preparing it in your instant pot at home.

TIME: 30 MINUTE | **SERVINGS:** 6

INGREDIENTS

6 Cups whole milk

Spices: 1 lemon peel (washed), $\frac{1}{2}$ tbsp vanilla extract, 6 tbsp cornstarch, 8tbsp sugar (powdered)

8egg yolks

For garnish: cinnamon stick and ground cinnamon

METHOD

1. Set your instant pot to sauté mode.
2. Pour 5 cups of milk to the instant pot and heat the milk. Do not boil. Add the lemon peel and cinnamon stick.
3. Remove the milk from the instant pot and let rest for ten minutes.
4. In a separate bowl whisk together remaining milk and cornstarch ensuring cornstarch completely dissolves in the milk.
5. In another bowl beat the egg yolks with sugar until frothy using your electric mixture. Add the cornstarch mixture and mix until well combined.
6. Us a slotted spoon to remove the lemon peel and cinnamon stick from the milk.
7. Return the milk to the instant pot and heat the milk. Do not let the milk boil. Add vanilla extract and the egg yolk mixture while stirring with the electric mixture.
8. Stir until the mixture thickens.
9. Pour the natillas into serving bowl s and refrigerate, sprinkle ground cinnamon and let cool. Enjoy.

INSTANT POT OATMEAL JARS

This is delicious, healthy, and gluten-free oatmeal jars to take as your snack or for breakfast. The oatmeal is easy to prepare in your instant pot and are all you need for your snack.

TIME: 15 MINUTES | **SERVINGS:** 5

INGREDIENTS

3 cups coconut or almond milk

Cereals: $1\frac{1}{4}$ cup rolled oats (gluten-free), $\frac{1}{2}$ Cup walnuts (chopped), $\frac{1}{4}$ Cup flaxseed

$\frac{1}{2}$ Cup apple (chopped)

1 carrot (shredded)

$\frac{1}{2}$ Cup cinnamon

METHOD

1. Pour the milk in the instant pot then the rolled oats.
2. Add all other ingredients and mix until well incorporated.
3. Set time for nine minutes .when time has elapsed let rest for two minutes then release pressure quickly.
4. Mix in a third cup of dairy cream and any optional protein.
5. Spoon the oatmeal into five serving bowls or mason jars then top with goji berries
6. You may also add a honey splash of milk, and a pinch of cinnamon.

NUTRITIONAL INFORMATION

Cal: 295 | Fat: 14g | Carbs: 32g | Fiber: 7g | Protein: 6.6g

CREAM CATALANA

Are you in search of an awesomely delicious dessert for your family or friends for your celebration event? This is creamy, sweet Mediterranean dessert will melt your mouth, and it's all you would ask for in a dessert.

TIME: 20 MINUTES | **SERVING:** 4

INGREDIENTS

4 egg yolks

1 cup sugar

Spices: 1 stick cinnamon, $\frac{1}{2}$ Lemon rind (grated)

1 tbsp cornstarch

2 cups milk

METHOD

1. Turn to sauté function on your instant pot on.
2. Beat egg yolks and three-quarter cup of sugar until frothy in your instant pot.
3. Add cinnamon and the lemon rind. Add cornstarch while stirring constantly.
4. Heat until the mixture thickens to your desired consistency.
5. Put off the instant pot. The mixture will curdle.
6. Your crema catalama is ready. Pour in four ramekins then refrigerate for three hours.
7. Sprinkle the remaining sugar on each ramekin and put the cream in a hot broiler until the sugar caramelizes
8. Serve and enjoy.

FRIXUELOS DE ASTURIAS RECIPE

These are yummy easy to make Austrian crepes which is a Hit in most homes on the Mediterranean diet. Serve these insanely addictive crepes and be assured of no leftovers in your house.

TIME: 15 MINUTES | **SERVING:** 12 FRIXUELOS

INGREDIENTS

2 tbsp butter

$1\frac{1}{2}$ Cup sifted flour

Seasonings: 3 tbsp sugar, $\frac{1}{2}$ tbsp salt

3 eggs

16 oz. milk

METHOD

1. Set your instant pot to sauté function on.
2. Place butter in the instant pot and let it melt. Do not let the butter burn.
3. In a mixing bowl whisk together flour, sugar, and salt. Set aside.
4. In another mixing bowl beat eggs until thick. Beat in the milk and the butter.
5. Add the wet ingredients into the dry mixture.
6. Add a small amount of butter in the instant pot and pour the batter using a ladle. Cook until browned on both sides.
7. Transfer into a warm plate and spoon filling of your choice at the Centre. You may use apple sauce, cream fruit preserves or egg custard.
8. Enjoy.

INSTANT POT YOGHURT

Are your kids yogurt lovers? Do you own an instant pot? If the answer to the questions is yes, then this yogurt is for you. It's creamier, cheaper and above all addictively delicious.

TIME: 8 HOURS | **SERVING:** 6

INGREDIENTS

8 cups whole milk

$\frac{1}{2}$ Cup plain whole milk yogurt

METHOD

1. Add milk into your instant pot .lid the instant pot and turn on the yogurt function.
2. Set pressure to boil and time for one hour.
3. When time is done cool the instant pot insert, you can place the instant pot insert in a bowl of cold water until milk reaches 100°F. Set aside a cup of milk.
4. In a mixing bowl whisk the reserved milk and the half cup of yogurt.
5. Stir in the yogurt mixture into the remaining milk.
6. Return the insert to the instant pot and turn on the yogurt function .set time for eight hours.
7. Transfer the yogurt to storage containers and let cool. Store up to 10 days.

EASY SPANISH BREAD PUDDING RECIPE

This sweet and easy to prepare Spanish bread is a Hit in the Mediterranean lifestyle. This side dish can also be taken as a filling breakfast. If this bread cools, it can be reheated using a toaster oven

TIME: 20 MINUTES | **SERVING:** 6

INGREDIENTS

6 bread slices

$\frac{3}{4}$ Cup milk

1 egg

Corn or canora oil

OPTIONAL

$\frac{1}{8}$ tbsp vanilla extract, $\frac{1}{4}$ Cup cinnamon sugar to sprinkle

METHOD

1. In a mixing bowl, pour milk then beat in the eggs. Add vanilla extract.
2. Set your instant pot at sauté mode and pour the vegetable oil such that the bottom is covered. Ensure the oil doesn't burn.
3. Place a slice of bread in the egg mixture and quickly place it in the instant pot. Ensure you don't soak the bread for a long time.
4. Repeat with each bread slice and cook on both sides. Place the bread slices on a plate and sprinkle cinnamon sugar
5. Drizzle honey and fresh fruits. Serve and enjoy.

PEACHES IN WINE

A peach in wine is a super delicious fresh dessert to finish that awesome dinner. Peaches have summer taste while the wine gives your dessert its zing. You can make this dessert ahead of time and store in the fridge.

TIME: 45 MINUTES | **SERVING:** 4

INGREDIENTS

4 firm peaches (ripe and peeled)

3 cups red wine

6tbsp sugar

4 tbsp brandy

METHOD

1. Pour the red wine, sugar, and brandy in a mixing bowl and stir until the sugar completely dissolves.
2. Set your instant pot to sauté mode. Fit in the peaches well in the instant pot. Pour the wine mixture into the instant pot.
3. Add cinnamon mixture and water to cover the peaches. Lid the instant pot and set time for fifteen minutes on steaming function. Let the wine boil.
4. When the time has elapsed release pressure naturally. Remove peaches from the instant pot and let cool at room temperature.
5. Remove the cinnamon stick and change the instant pot setting to sauté mode. Let the liquid boil making the syrup more intense in flavor.
6. Allow liquid to cool and pour it over the peaches. Serve and enjoy with a scoop of vanilla ice cream

NUTRITIONAL INFORMATION

Cal: 266| Fat: 0g| Carbs: 34g| Fiber: 2g| Protein: 1g| Sugar: 0g

INSTANT POT ITALIAN PASTA

Are you sometimes in a time crunch? This instant pot Italian pasta is a classic, quick, ready in five minutes dish that will make yourself and your family go nuts. This pasta will keep you full until the next meal. You definitely need to try this dish.

TIME: 10 MINUTES | **SERVING:** 3

INGREDIENTS

1 lb. Italian sausage

1 lb. penne pasta

Seasonings: 1 tbsp Italian seasoning,

Liquids: 24 oz. marinara, 2 cups chicken broth, whipping cream

Parmesan (freshly shredded)

METHOD

1. Switch your instant pot to sauté mode and cook the sausage until well cooked. Turn the instant pot off.
2. Spread the cooked sausage at the bottom of the instant pot and pour penne pasta over the cooked sausage. Sprinkle Italian seasoning on the pasta.
3. Pour marinara over the pasta followed by the chicken broth. Do not stir.
4. Lid the instant pot and set time for five minutes on high pressure. When the time has elapsed release pressure quickly.
5. Stir in the desired amount of whipping cream.
6. Serve pasta and top with fresh parmesan.

SWEET AND SALTY SPANISH PEANUTS

If your kids are peanuts lovers, no need to visit the restaurant again. Just grab your instant pot, and you can now enjoy more appetizing and cheap sweet and salty peanuts from your home.

TIME: 20 MINUTES | **SERVING:** 2

INGREDIENTS

1 tbsp oil

1 Lb. Spanish peanuts (raw)

Salt and pepper to taste

1 tbsp sugar

METHOD

1. Set your instant pot to sauté mod.
2. Heat oil then add the peanuts. Add salt and pepper to taste.
3. Stir cook peanuts until browned. Turn off the instant pot when then peanuts are cooked.
4. Add sugar and mix until well incorporated.
5. Remove the peanuts from the instant pot and let cool. Serve and enjoy.

INSTANT POT CHICKEN SHAWARMA

Are you an instant pot fan? These chicken shawarma will blow your taste buds away. Instead of ordering them from your favorite restaurant just make them at home in your instant pot.

TIME: 35 MINUTES | **SERVING:** 5

1 lb. chicken breasts and chicken thighs (boneless, skinless, and sliced into strips)

Spices: 1 tbsp cumin (ground), 1 tbsp paprika, $\frac{1}{2}$ tbsp turmeric, $\frac{1}{4}$ tbsp garlic (granulated), $\frac{1}{4}$ tbsp allspice (ground), $\frac{1}{4}$ chili powder, $\frac{1}{8}$ tbsp cinnamon (ground)

Salt and pepper to taste

1 cup chicken broth

METHOD

1. Place the chicken breast and thighs in your instant pot.
2. In a mixing bowl combine all the spices then pour the spices over the chicken.
3. Add salt and pepper to taste. Mix the spices and the chicken such that it is well coated.
4. Add chicken broth and lid the instant pot. Put on the poultry setting on and time for fifteen minutes.
5. Once the time has elapsed, release pressure naturally for ten minutes.
6. Serve the chicken with veggies or on sweet potato toast. Drizzle tahini sauce.

Conclusion

Dear readers! It's time to say goodbye to you! But this is not the end, it is the beginning of your Mediterranean Diet Instant Pot cooking journey!

I think you must have already learned too much from this book! Now all you need to do is to try these delicious simple recipes!

Wish you a happy life!

APPENDIX: MEASUREMENT CHART

LIQUID VOLUME MEASUREMENTS

U.S. Liquid Volume Measurements

Cups	Fluid Ounces	Tablespoons	Teaspoons
1	8	16	48
3/4	6	12	36
1/2	4	8	24
1/3	2 2/3	5 tbsp + 1 tsp	16
1/4	2	4	12
1/16	.5	1	3

WEIGHT CONVERSIONS

Weight Conversions

Imperial	Metric
1/2 oz.	14 g
1 oz.	28 g
2 oz.	57 g
3 oz.	85 g
4 oz.	113 g
5 oz.	142 g
6 oz.	170 g
7 oz.	199 g
8 oz.	227 g
9 oz.	255 g
10 oz.	284 g
12 oz	340 g
1 lb.	454 g
1 ½ lb.	680 g
2 lb.	907 g
2.2 lb.	1 kg

LIQUID VOLUME CONVERSION

Liquid Volume Conversions

Fluid Ounces	Cups	Milliliters	Liters
2	1/4	59	.059
4	1/2	118	.118
8	1	237	.237
16	2	473	.473
24	3	710	.71
32	4	946	.946
33.6	4.22	1000	1

METRIC TEMPERATURE CONVERSIONS

Temperature Conversions

Fahrenheit	Celsius	Gas Mark	Description
225	107	1/4	Very Low
250	121	1/2	Very Low
275	135	1	Low
300	149	2	Low
325	163	3	Moderate
350	177	4	Moderate
375	190	5	Moderately Hot
400	204	6	Moderately Hot
425	218	7	Hot
450	238	8	Hot
475	246	9	Very Hot

Made in the USA
Middletown, DE
18 February 2020

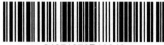